AF270582

MY FRIEND WITH ALLERGIES

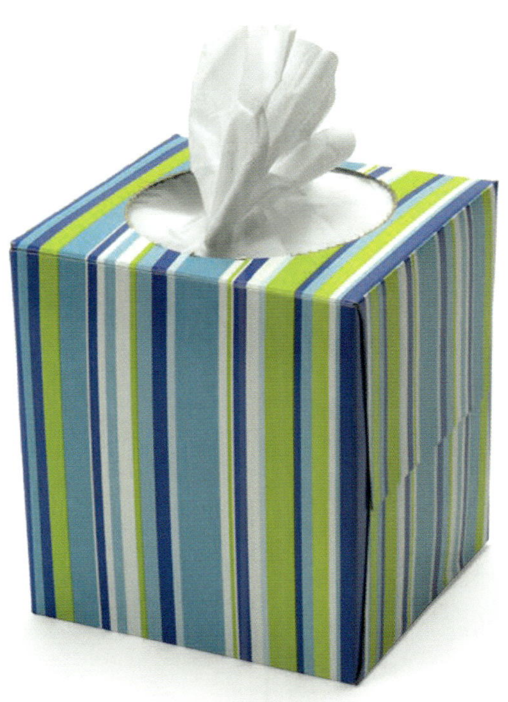

by Elizabeth Andrews

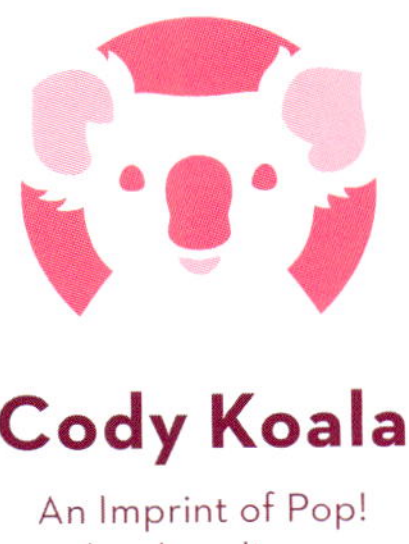

Cody Koala

An Imprint of Pop!
popbooksonline.com

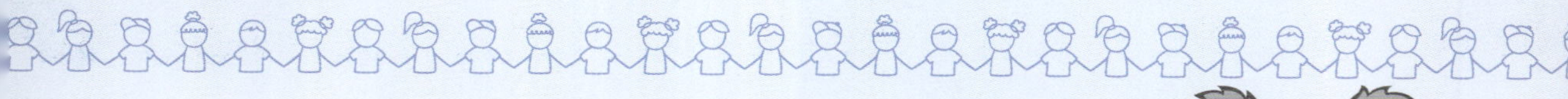

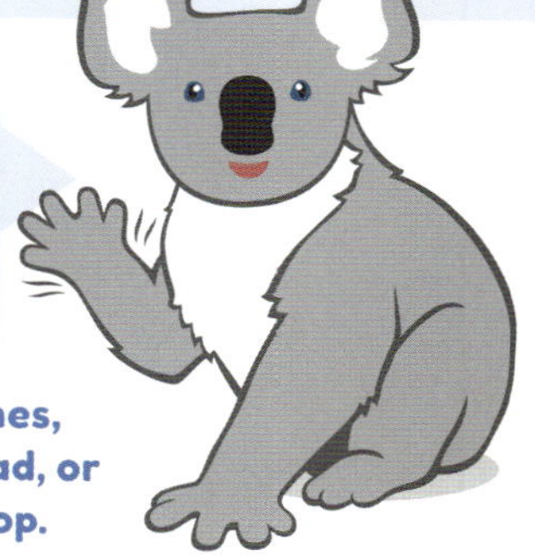

Hello! My name is
Cody Koala

This book is filled with videos, puzzles, games, and more! Scan the QR codes* while you read, or visit the website below to make this book pop.

popbooksonline.com/allergies

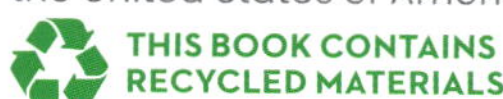

*Scanning QR codes requires a web-enabled smart device with a QR code reader app and a camera.

abdobooks.com

Published by Pop!, a division of ABDO, PO Box 398166, Minneapolis, Minnesota 55439. Copyright ©2024 by Abdo Consulting Group, Inc. International copyrights reserved in all countries. No part of this book may be reproduced in any form without written permission from the publisher. Cody Koala™ is a trademark and logo of Pop!.

Printed in the United States of America, North Mankato, Minnesota.
102023
012024

THIS BOOK CONTAINS RECYCLED MATERIALS

Cover Photo: Shutterstock Images
Interior Photos: Shutterstock Images; Getty Images
Editor: Grace Hansen
Series Designer: Victoria Bates

Library of Congress Control Number: 2023938794

Publisher's Cataloging-in-Publication Data
Names: Andrews, Elizabeth, author.
Title: My friend with allergies / by Elizabeth Andrews
Description: Minneapolis, Minnesota : Pop!, 2024 | Series: My friend with health needs | Includes online resources and index
Identifiers: ISBN 9781098245283 (lib. bdg.) | ISBN 9781098245849 (ebook)
Subjects: LCSH: Friendship--Juvenile literature. | Allergies--Juvenile literature. | Allergy in children--Juvenile literature. | Social acceptance--Juvenile literature.
Classification: DDC 616.202--dc23

Table of Contents

Chapter 1
Feeling Sneezy! 4

Chapter 2
What Are Allergies? 6

Chapter 3
Taking Care of Allergies . . . 10

Chapter 4
In an Emergency 16

Making Connections 22
Glossary 23
Index 24
Online Resources 24

Feeling Sneezy!

Maddy loves flowers. But when she's in the garden, her eyes itch and her nose runs. Maddy's mom gives her medicine. It helps Maddy enjoy the outdoors!

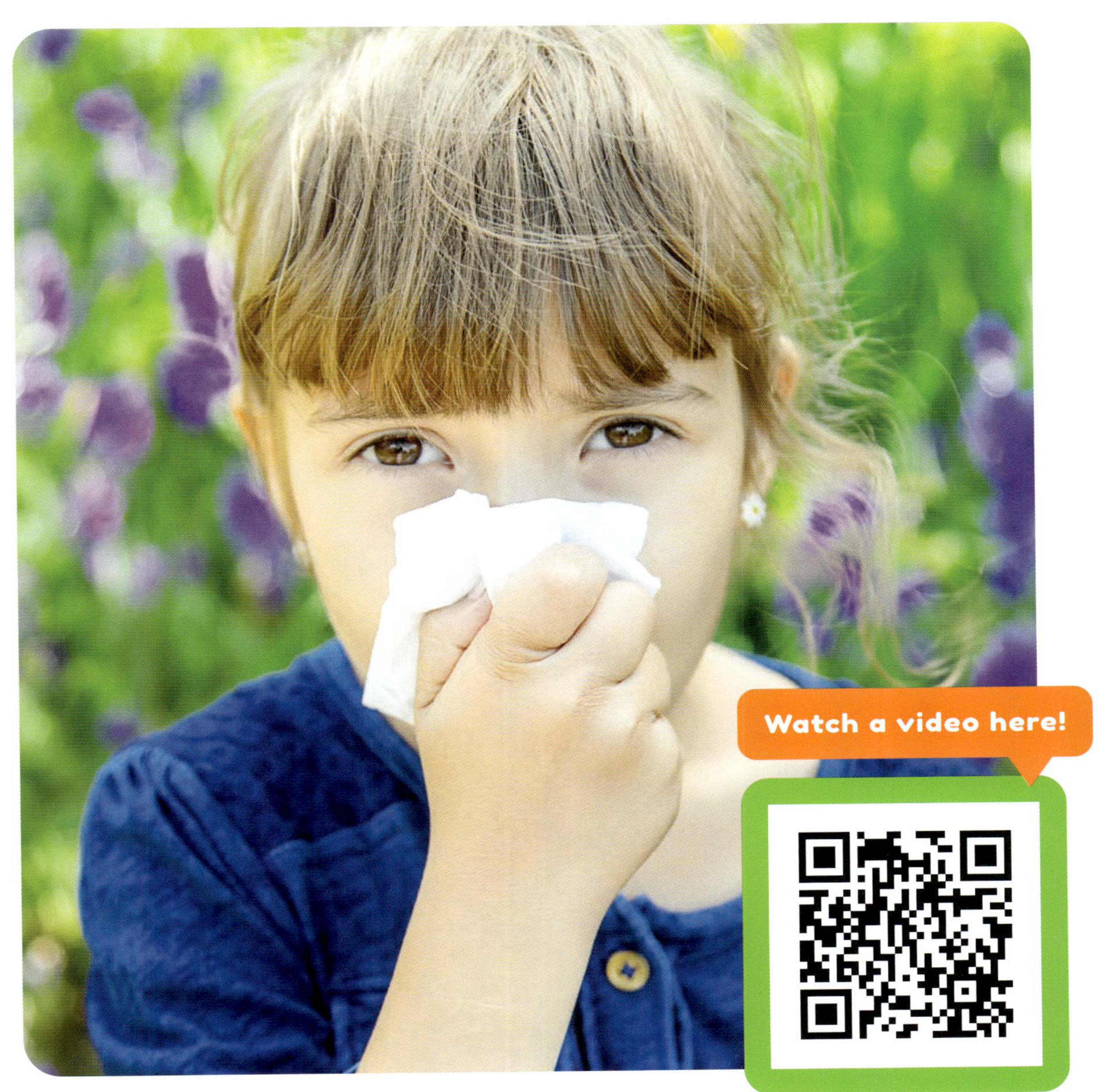
Watch a video here!

Chapter 2

What Are Allergies?

A person has allergies because their body mistakes common **substances** as harmful. These things are called allergens.

Common Allergies

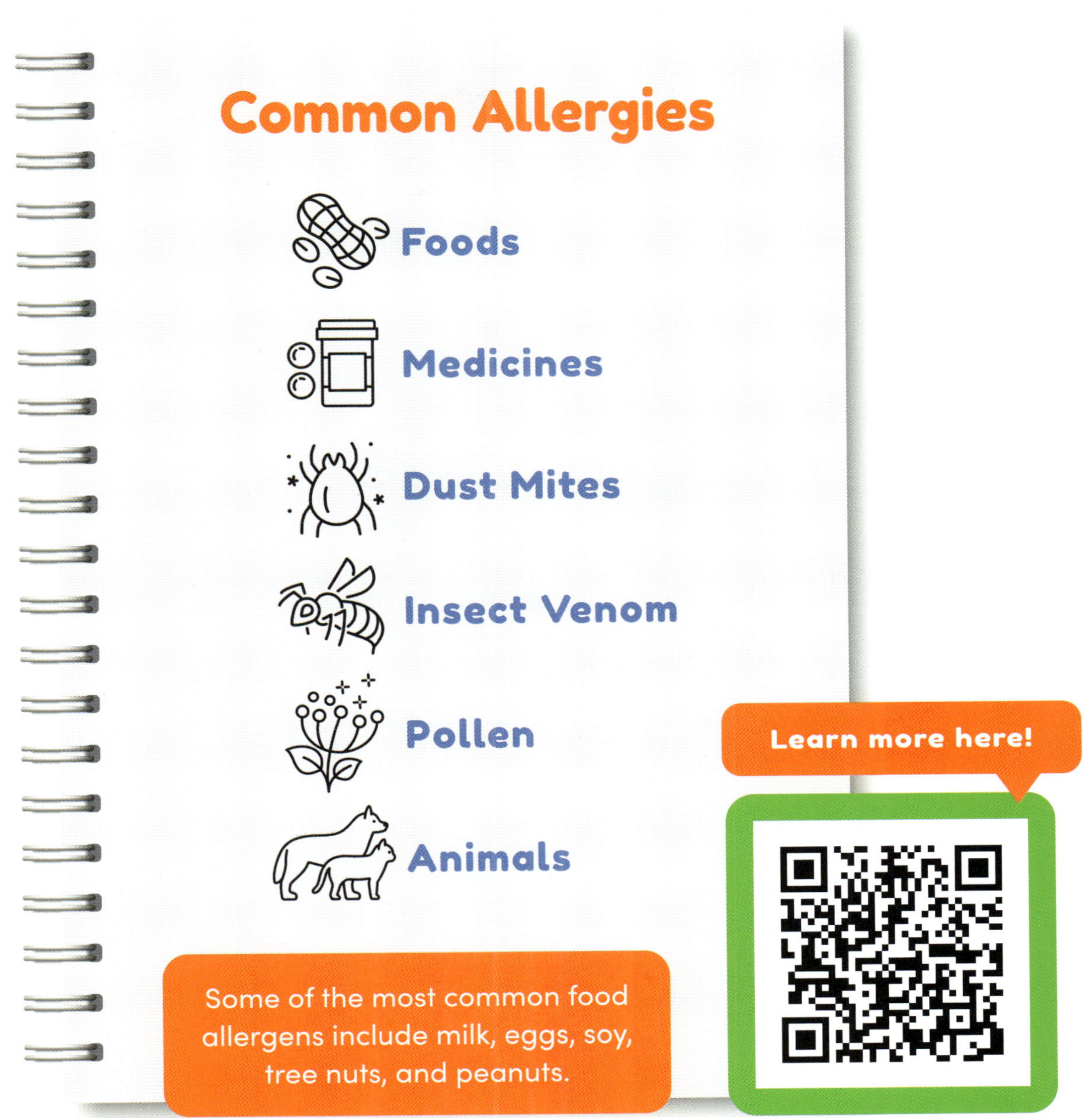

- Foods
- Medicines
- Dust Mites
- Insect Venom
- Pollen
- Animals

Some of the most common food allergens include milk, eggs, soy, tree nuts, and peanuts.

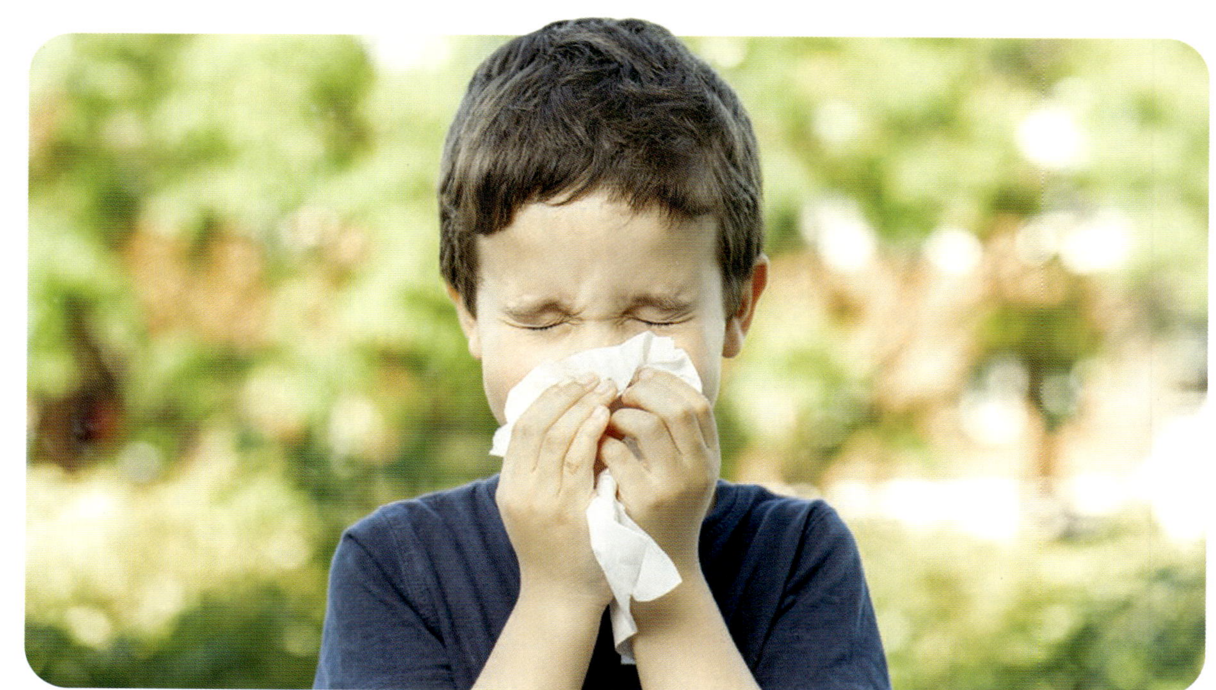

When the body thinks
something is harmful,
it will try to get it out by
releasing histamines.

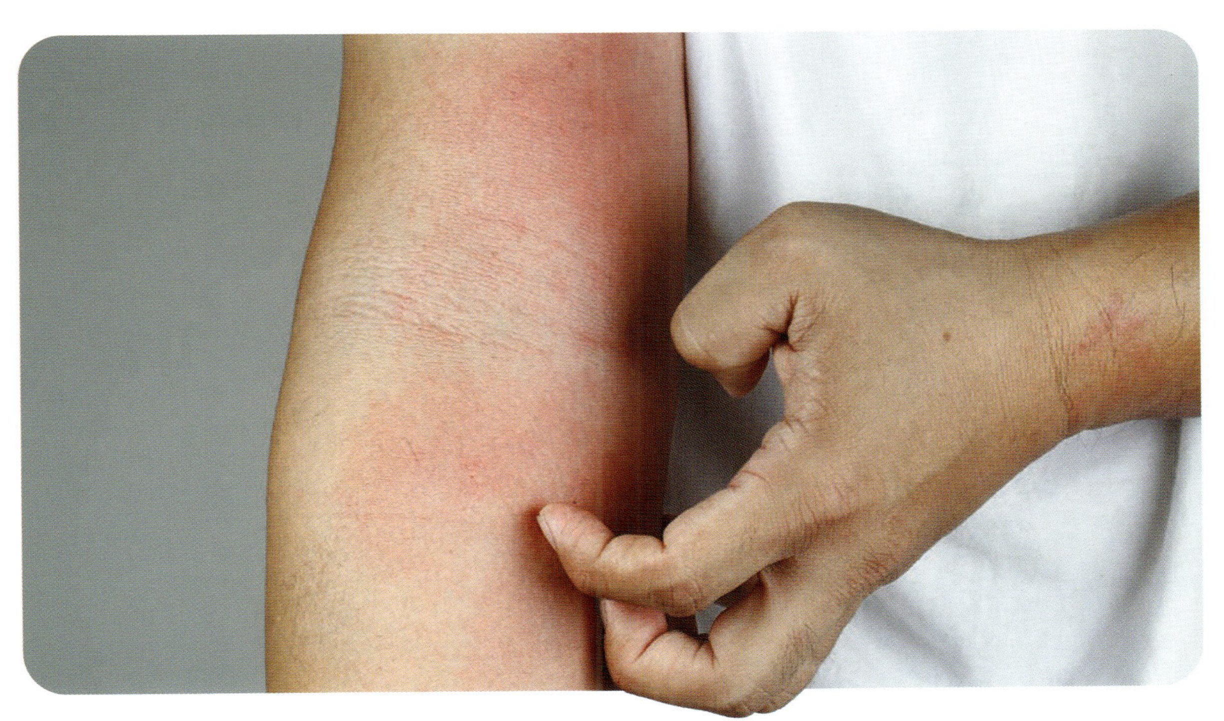

Histamines cause allergic

reactions, such as a runny

nose, red eyes, coughing,

and **hives**.

Chapter 3

Taking Care of Allergies

The best way to take care of allergies is by **avoiding** the allergen. If someone is allergic to peanuts, they should not eat them. If someone is allergic to dogs, they should not pet them.

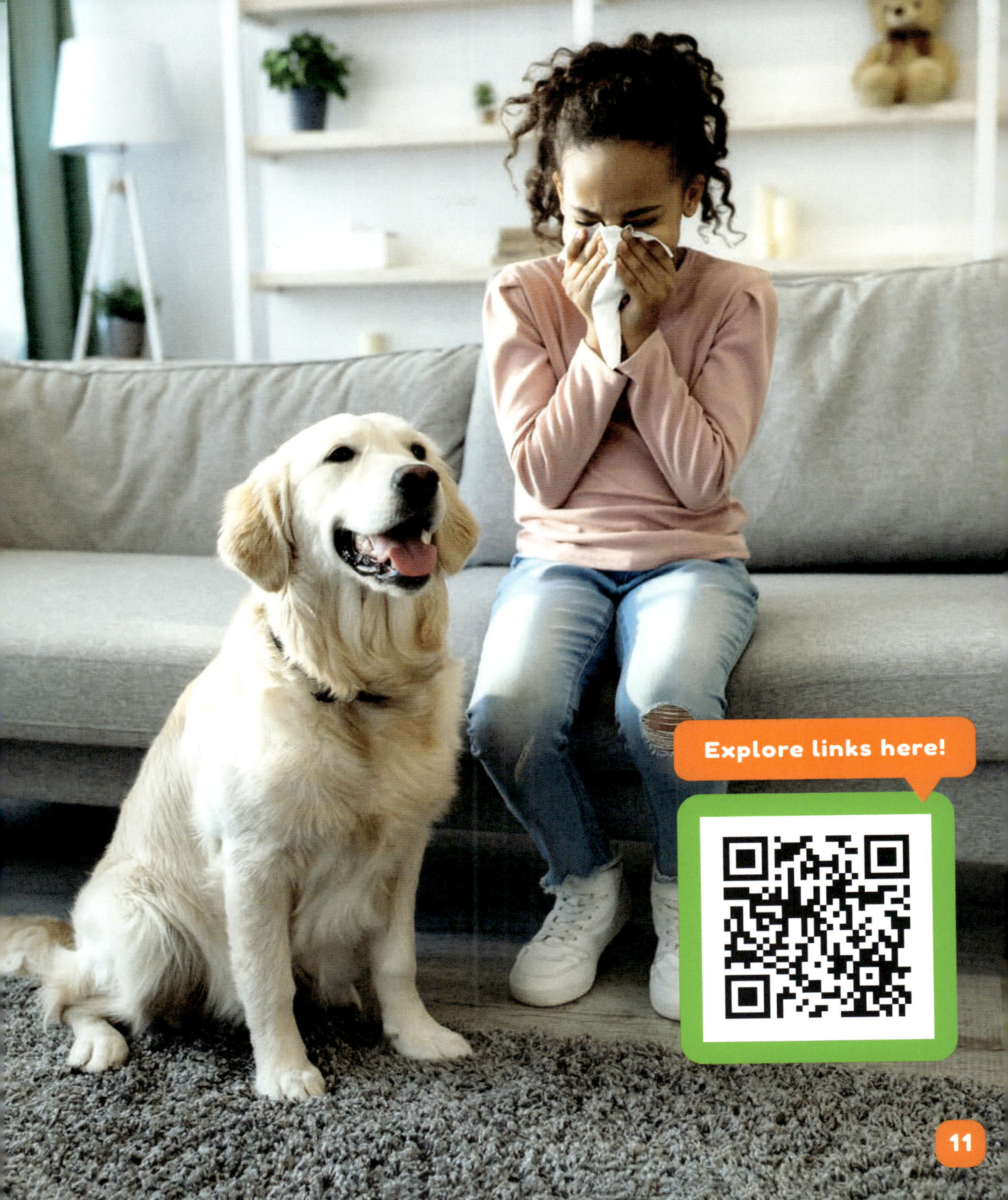
Explore links here!

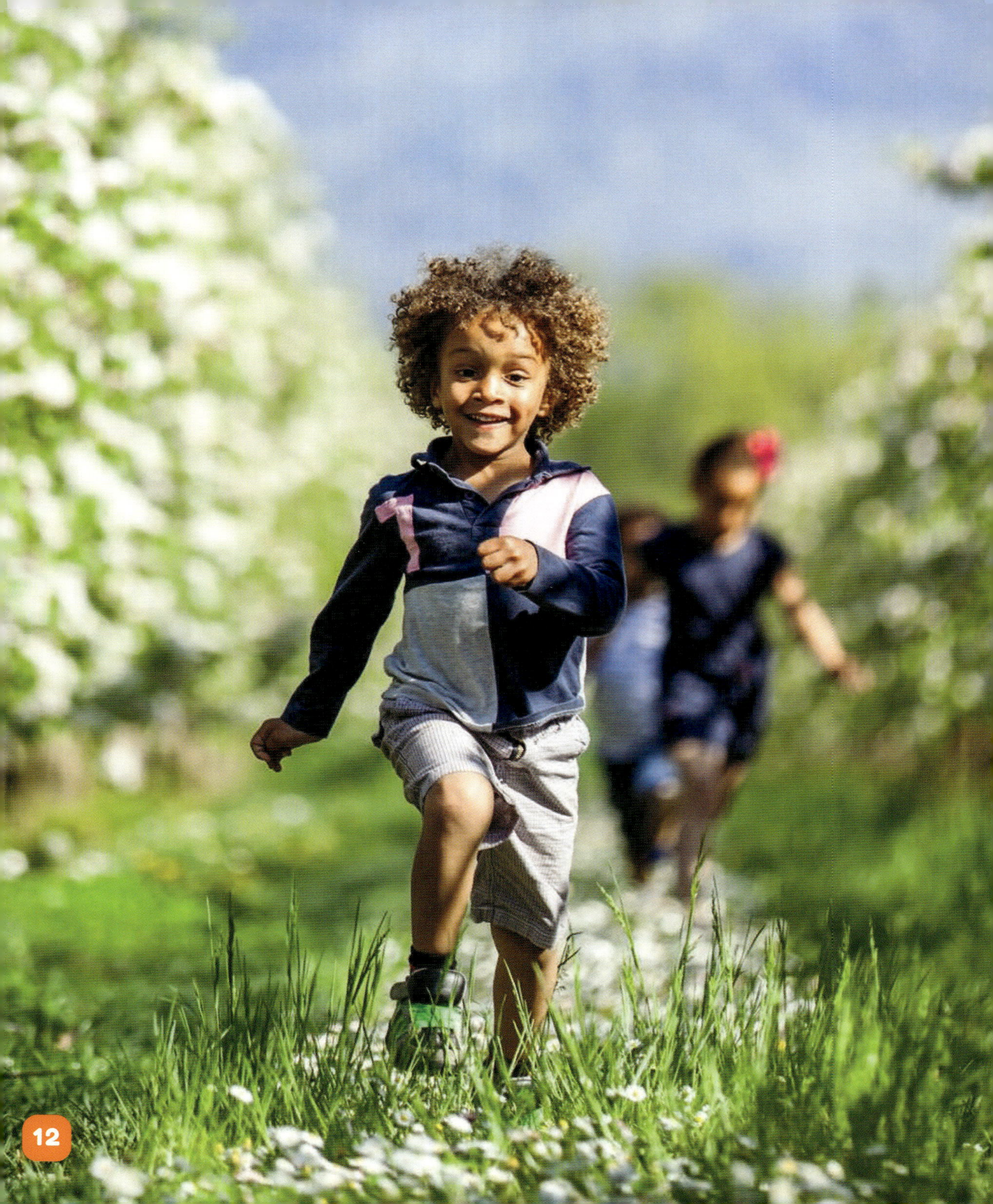

Some allergies are troublesome but can be **managed** easily. People who are allergic to **pollen** can't avoid it in the springtime. But they can take medicine.

Sometimes, allergic

reactions can be dangerous.

A person might throw

up or break out in **hives**.

They could have difficulty

breathing or a racing

heartbeat. These kinds of

reactions are **emergencies**.

Some people with food allergies find it safer to cook at home. This way, they can control the ingredients.

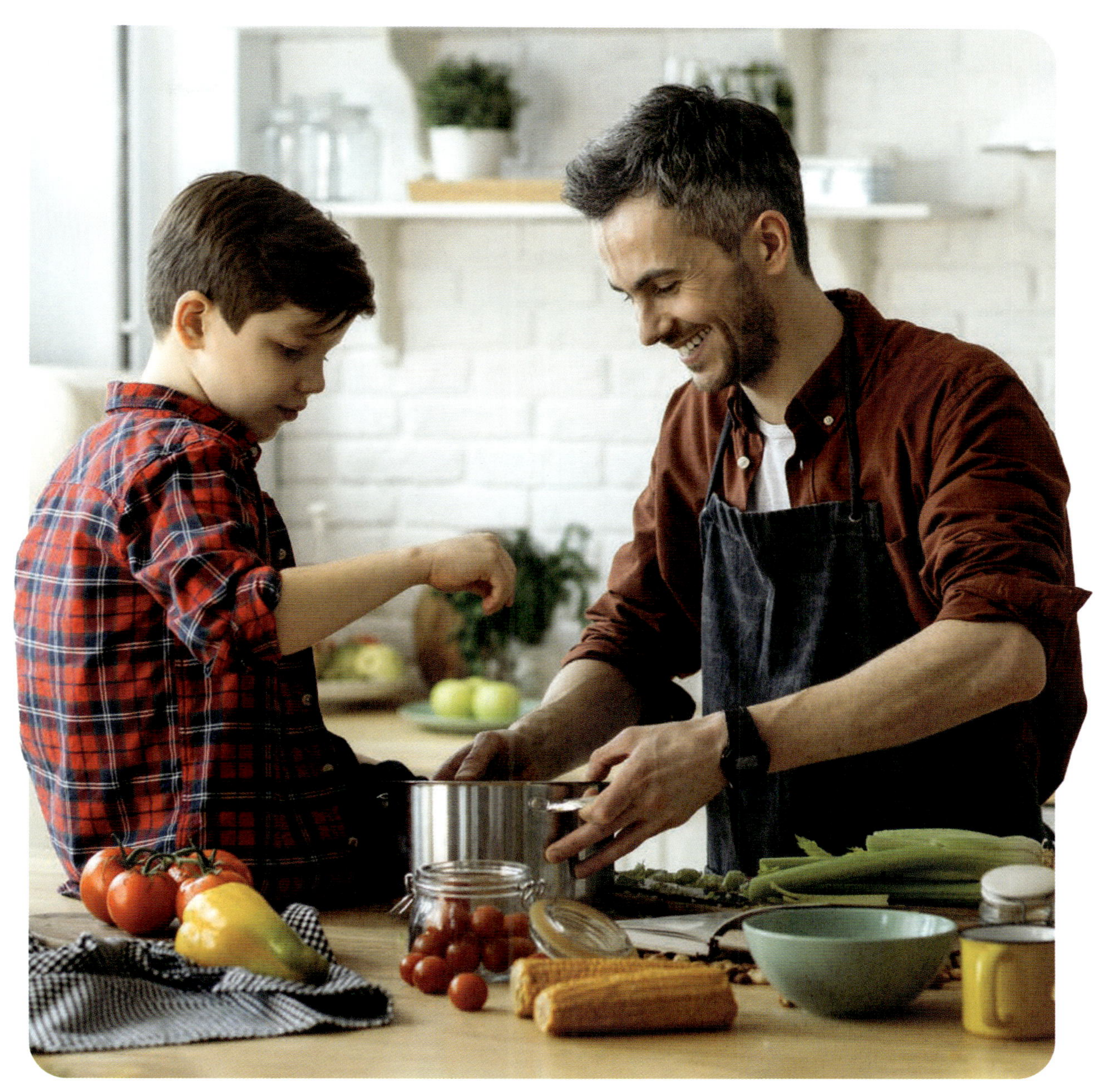

Chapter 4

In an Emergency

A person having a **severe** allergic **reaction** often needs to use an EpiPen. Then they need to go to the **emergency** room. These reactions are usually caused by food or insect bites and stings.

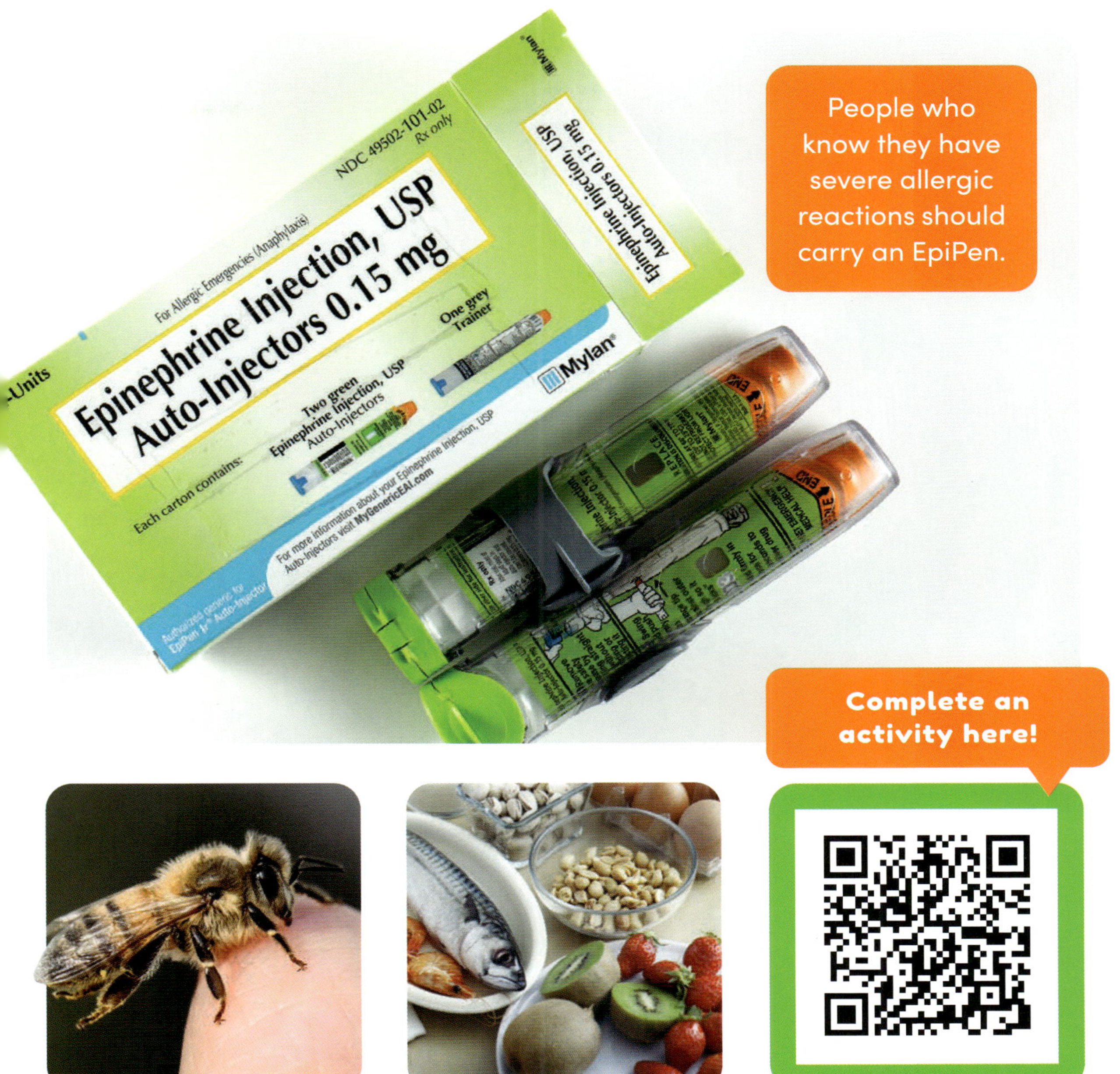
People who know they have severe allergic reactions should carry an EpiPen.
Complete an activity here!

Food allergies can be

the most harmful. They

are important to **avoid**.

For example, people who

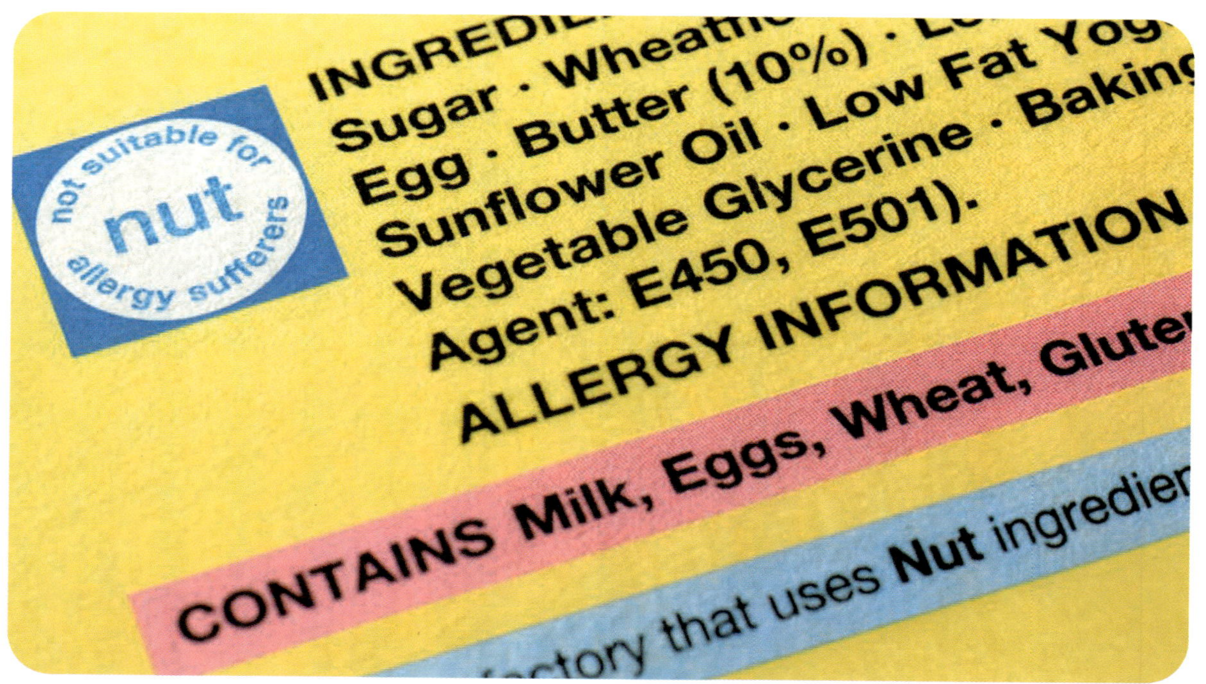

are allergic to peanuts
make sure to look at the
ingredients list before they
eat a food item.

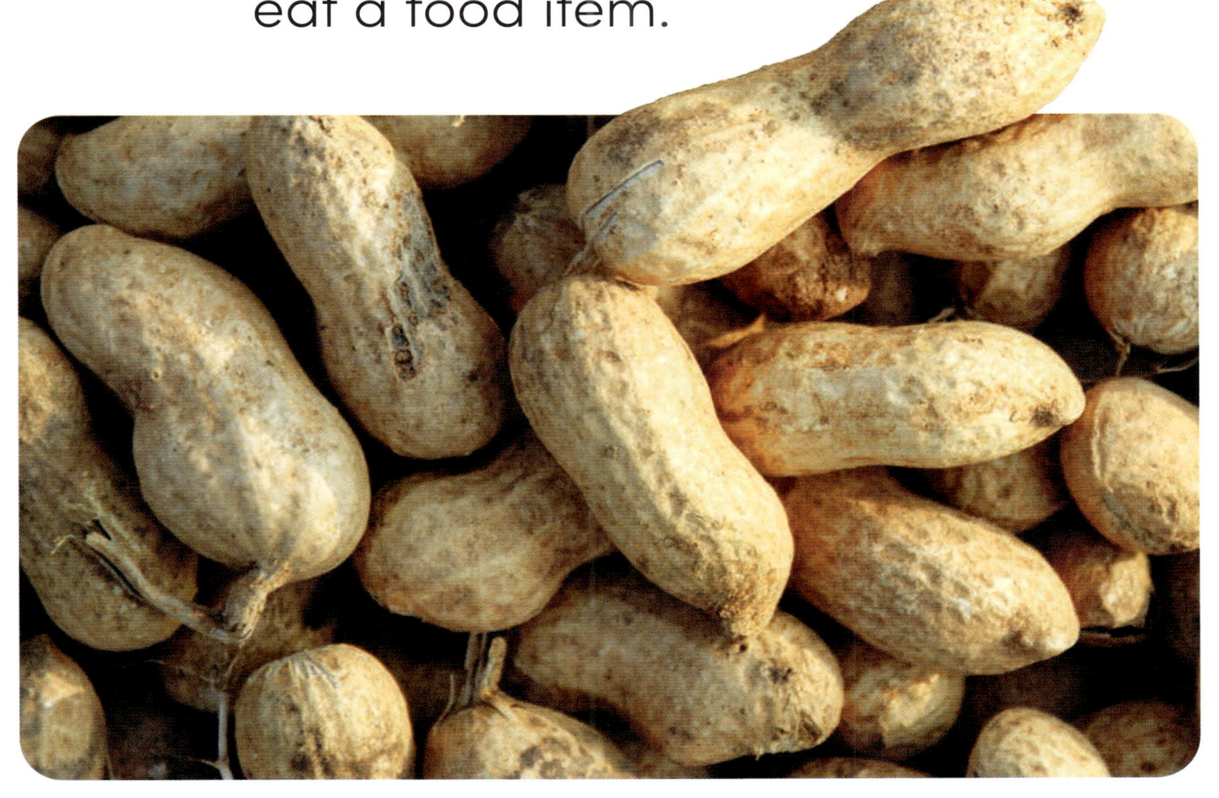

Many children have allergies. No one's allergies are exactly the same. But if people safely **manage** their allergies, they can enjoy life just like their friends!

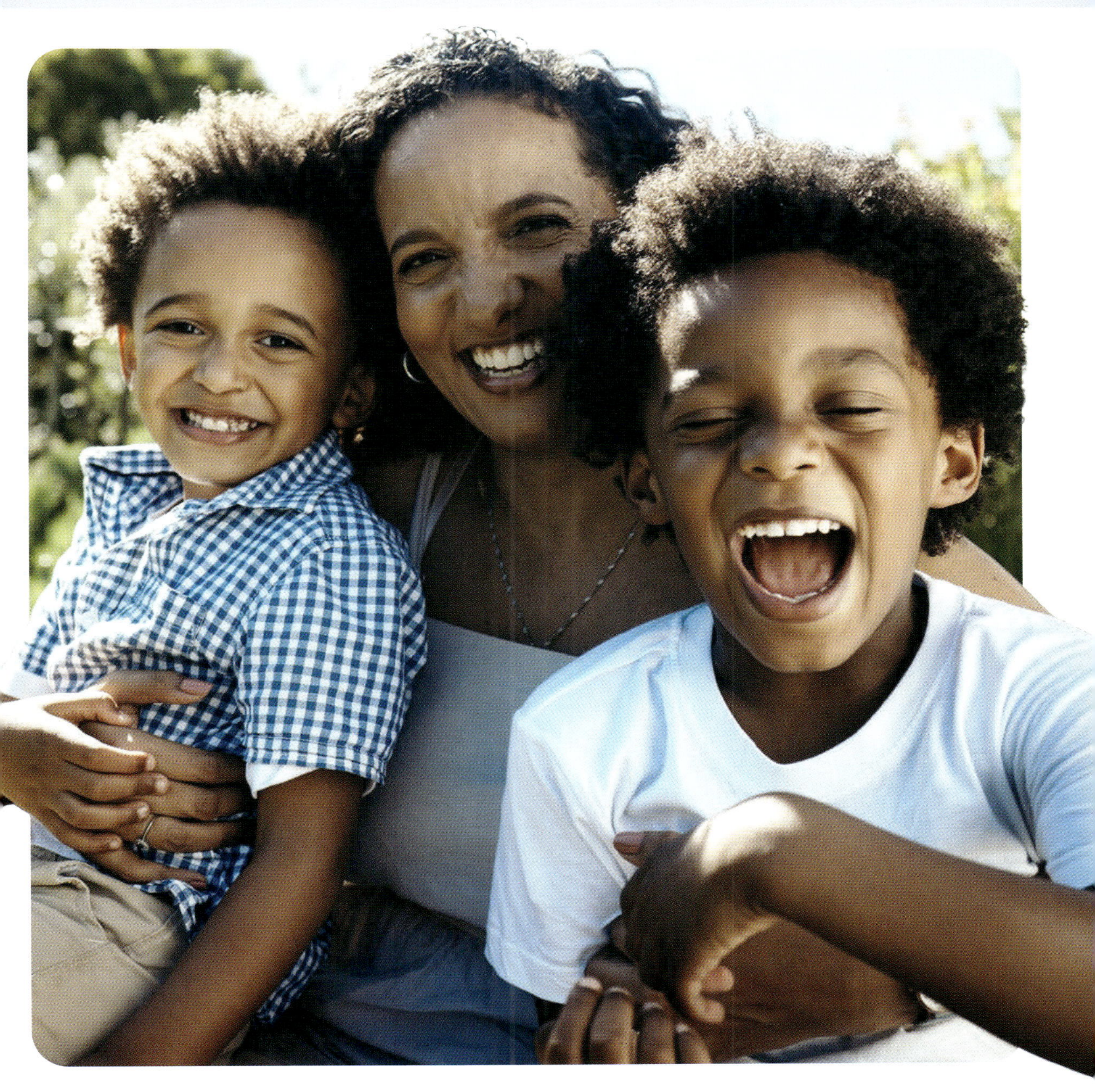

Making Connections

Text-to-Self

Do you have any allergies? If so, how do you manage them?

Text-to-Text

Have you read any books about other kinds of health needs? If so, how were they similar to or different from having allergies?

Text-to-World

What small changes could the world make so that things are safer for people with serious allergies?

Glossary

avoid – to keep away from.

emergency – an unexpected event that requires immediate action.

hive – red, itchy, and swollen areas on the skin.

manage – to look after or make decisions about.

pollen – the fine, yellow powder made by a flowering plant.

reaction – the body's physical response to an allergen.

severe – very strong or intense.

substance – a particular kind of matter.

Index

allergens, 6–7, 10

animals, 7, 10, 16

EpiPen, 16

foods, 7, 10, 16, 18–19

histamines, 8–9

medicine, 4, 7, 13

pollen, 7, 13

reactions, 4, 9, 14, 16

severe reactions, 14, 16

Online Resources

popbooksonline.com

Thanks for reading this Cody Koala book!

This book is filled with videos, puzzles, games, and more! Scan the QR codes* while you read, or visit the website below to make this book pop.

popbooksonline.com/allergies

*Scanning QR codes requires a web-enabled smart device with a QR code reader app and a camera.